Keto Slow Cooker Cookbook

Burn your fat with delicious low carb recipes. Enjoy rich nutrient food cooked at low temterature.

Marion Gambini

© Copyright 2021 - All rights reserved.

TABLE OF CONTENTS

Introduction

Going on a keto diet means you have to cook most of your meals at home, as most foods served in eating places are not keto-friendly. Many of us have a day-job so that cooking may become a chore. After you come home exhausted from a day's work, the thought of cooking is not a pleasant one. So, the slow cooker comes to the rescue to who wants and wishes to eat nutritious Keto meals can now come home with food ready to eat. While you are working at the office or doing other chores, cooking your food will be unattended in your kitchen with the magic of your slow cooker. The fantastic slow cooker allows you to prepare the ingredients in the morning and have it ready for lunch or dinner. Or you can even let it cook while you sleep so you can wake up to an excellent ready breakfast. You can even pack some of it for your lunch at work.

For example, you can cook your favorite pulled pork overnight to supply the meat needed for a keto-friendly wrap using lettuce or omelet and packed it as your lunch after you had your breakfast. Or you can make meatballs during the day and save some for breakfast (freeze in your fridge after cooking) for the next morning. For it to make even more time saving, many ingredients can be prepared the night before. Chopped the necessary ingredients, put them in airtight containers of Ziploc bags, and stored in the fridge overnight to speed things along in the morning. In the morning, before you leave work, pour the ingredients into the pot out and turn on your slow cooker and start cooking. Hence, the slow cooker is an indispensable cooking gadget for those doing the keto diet.

Other benefits that the slow cooker will provide you are:

Save Electricity: Compared to the oven, the slow-cooker uses less electricity. On low, it runs on the same amount of energy needed to power a 75 to a 100-watt light bulb. Lower heat production: Your house is not going to get warm, unlike using an oven, and you don't have to fear that your house will burn down due to overheating. The slow-cooker is safe to leave to its own devices without any supervision, unlike dishes left in the oven or on the stovetop. More meat choices: You can now include tougher meat on your menu. The slow, moist cooking environment breaks the tough tissue of less tender, but very affordable, cuts of meat—the portions of muscle used the most, such as the chuck, brisket, round, and shank. It is perfect for cooking lamb shanks! High nutritious food: The slow-cooking of bones and meats melt collagens that enrich the dish's liquid with its flavor and many nutrients. It is perfect for making healthy and delicious soups.

In this cookbook, we will go in-depth first with Keto history and how it works, then we will get to know your slow cooker and how to use it, and finally, we will provide you 200 Keto-friendly recipes that will surely bring your slow cooker at its best.

CHAPTER 1:

Breakfast

1. Keto Slow Cooker Tasty Onions

Preparation time: 15 minutes

Cooking time: 6 hours

Servings: 4

Ingredients:

- 4 (or 5) large pcs onions, sliced

- 4 tablespoon butter or coconut oil

- 1/4 cup coconu aminos

- Splenda (optional)

- Salt and pepper

Directions: Place the onion slices into the Slow CookerTop the onion slices with coconut amino and butter; you might add Splenda at will.

1. Cook it on low during 6-7 hours. Serve over the grilled vegetables.**Nutrition:**Calories: 38 Carbs: 9g Fat: 0g Protein: 0g

2. Slow Cooker Benedict Casserole

Preparation time: 15 minutes

Cooking time: 4 hours

Servings: 7

Ingredients:

For the Casserole

- 1 large English muffin, cut into portions

- 1 lb. Canadian bacon, thick-cut

- 10 large eggs

- 1 cup milk

- salt and pepper

For the Sauce

- 6 egg yolks

- 1 1/2 tablespoon lemon juice

- 1 1/2 sticks unsalted butter, melted

- salt

- pinch of cayenne

Directions:

1. For the muffin: Using a medium-sized skillet, melt the butter. Add coconut and almond flour, egg, salt, and stir everything well. Add baking soda. Grease the Slow Cooker with cooking spray. Pour the mixture, put on low for 2 hours. Remove once done.

2. Grease again the Slow Cooker with cooking spray, cut the muffin into equal pieces, put on the bottom.

3. Slice the bacon, sprinkle half of it over top of the muffin pieces.

4. Whisk milk, eggs, season with salt and black pepper in a large bowl.

5. Pour the egg batter evenly over the muffin pieces and top with the rest of the bacon.

6. Cook on low within 2 hours in the slow cooker. Remove, and keep the muffins covered before serving.

7. To make the sauce, set up a double boiler, put the egg yolks, squeeze lemon juice in a bowl, and mix.

8. Put your bowl over the double boiler, continue whisking carefully; the bowl mustn't get too hot.

9. Put in the melted butter while continuing to whisk.

10. Season with salt and pepper. You may also add a little bit more lemon juice or cayenne.

11. Serve and enjoy.

Nutrition:

Calories: 286

Carbs: 16g

Fat: 19g

Protein: 14g

3. Crustless Slow Cooker Spinach Quiche

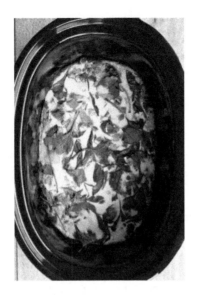

Preparation time: 15 minutes

Cooking time: 2 hours

Servings: 11

Ingredients:

- 10 oz. package frozen spinach

- 1 tablespoon butter or ghee

- 1 medium red bell pepper

- 1 1/2 cups cheddar cheese

- 8 pcs eggs

- 1 cup homemade sour cream

- 2 tablespoons fresh chives

- 1/2 teaspoon sea salt

- 1/4 teaspoon ground black pepper

- 1/2 cup ground almond flour

- 1/4 teaspoon baking soda

Directions:

1. Let the frozen spinach thaw and drain it well. Chop finely. Wash the pepper and slice it. Remove the seeds. Grate the cheddar cheese and set aside. Chop the fresh chives finely. Grease the slow cooker with cooking spray. Take a little skillet, heat the butter over high heat on the stove, sauté the pepper until tender, for about 6 minutes. Mix the eggs, sour cream, salt, plus pepper in a large bowl. Add grated cheese and chives and continue to mix. In another medium-sized bowl, combine almond flour with baking soda. Pour into the egg mixture, add peppers to the egg's mixture, and pour gently into the slow cooker. Set to cook on high within 2 hours then Serve.

Nutrition: Calories: 153 Carbs: 19g Fat: 3g Protein: 9g

4. Broccoli Gratin with Parmesan and Swiss Cheese

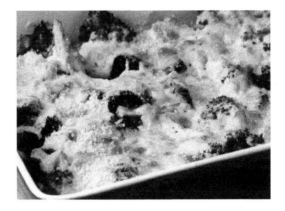

Preparation time: 15 minutes

Cooking time: 1 hour

Servings: 7

Ingredients:

- 8 cups bite-size broccoli flowerets

- 1 1/2 cups Swiss cheese

- 8 teaspoons mayo

- 1 1/2 tablespoon lemon juice

- 3/4 teaspoon Dijon mustard

- 3 tablespoons green onions

- 1/4 cup Parmesan cheese

- black pepper and salt to taste

Directions:

1. Wash broccoli and cut into small florets. Grate both parmesan and Swiss cheese into a bowl. Set aside.

2. Squeeze juice of a lemon into a cup. Wash and chop the green onions.

3. Grease with cooking spray or olive oil (optional) over the bottom of the slow cooker.

4. Put broccoli florets in a single layer. Mix in a separate bowl lemon juice, mustard, mayo, black pepper, add to the mixture green onion and grated cheese.

5. Put the mixture over the broccoli, cover, and cook on low 1 hour. Serve hot.

Nutrition:

Calories: 210 Carbs: 44g Fat: 2g

Protein: 5g

5. Slow Cooker Cream Cheese French Toast

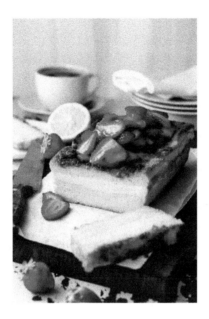

Preparation time: 15 minutes

Cooking time: 2 hours

Servings: 9

Ingredients:

- 1 (8-oz) package cream cheese

- ¼ cup slivered almonds

- 1 loaf keto bread

- 4 pcs eggs

- 1 teaspoon almond extract

- 1 tablespoon sweetener

- 1 cup milk

- 2 tablespoon butter

- ½ cup Cheddar cheese

- Maple syrup, at will, for dressing

Directions:

1. Mixcream cheese with almonds in a large bowl. Slice the keto bread into 2-inch slices. Try to make a 1/2-inch slit (horizontal) at the bottom of every piece to make a pocket.

2. Fill all the slices with cream mixture. Set aside. In a little bowl, mix eggs, extract the sweetener in milk. Coat the keto slices into the mix.

3. Grease with cooking spray the slow cooker over the bottom and sides, then put the coated keto slices on the slow cooker's base. Put on the top of each separate piece additional shredded cheese.

4. Cook on low for 2 hours. Serve hot.

Nutrition: Calories: 280

Carbs: 34g

Fat: 8g

Protein: 19g

6. Cheese and Sausage Breakfast

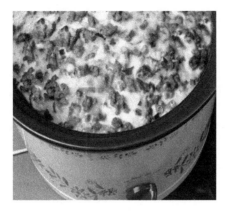

Preparation time: 15 minutes

Cooking time: 2 hours

Servings: 8

Ingredients:

- 2 tablespoon butter, softened

- 8 oz. breakfast sausage

- 1 lb. sweet potatoes, peeled and cubed

- 12 eggs

- 1 cup milk

- ¾ teaspoon salt

- ¼ teaspoon black pepper

- 4 oz. shredded mild cheddar cheese

Directions:

1. Coat the slow cooker and inside of the foil collar using softened butter.

2. Sauté in a large skillet over medium heat, the breakfast sausage until cooked through and browned, about 5 to 8 minutes.

3. Put the sweet potatoes into a microwave-safe bowl. Add 1 tablespoon water and cover bowl with a damp paper towel— microwave on high within 3 to 4 minutes.

4. Arrange the sausage and sweet potatoes in the bottom of the slow cooker.

5. Toss eggs, black pepper, milk, and salt to combine. Add the cheese; stir to mix very well.

6. Pour the egg/cheese mixture over sausage and sweet potatoes.

7. Then put 2 layers of paper towels below the slow cooker lid before.

8. Cook on high for 2 hours. Slice and serve.

Nutrition: Calories: 326 Carbs: 14g Protein: 18g

Fat: 22g Cholesterol: 291mg

Sodium: 650mg Potassium: 408mg Fiber: 2g

Sugar: 4g

7. Mushrooms, Cauliflower, and Zucchini Toast

Preparation time: 15 minutes

Cooking time: 7 hours

Servings: 8

Ingredients:

- 3-pound boneless beef chuck roast

- 2 cups keto compliant beef broth

- 5-7 radishes, cut into halves

- 1½ cups cauliflower florets

- ½ cup chopped celery

- 1/3 cup zucchini rounds

- ¼ cup chopped orange bell pepper

- 1 teaspoon xanthan gum (optional to thicken the gravy)

- 2 sprigs fresh rosemary

- Fresh parsley (for garnish)

- 1 teaspoon Himalayan sea salt

- ½ teaspoon freshly ground black pepper

- 1 teaspoon garlic powder

- ½ teaspoon dried Italian seasoning

- 1 tablespoon avocado oil or ghee

- 1 small onion chopped

- ½ cup sliced mushrooms

- 1 tablespoon tomato paste

- 1 teaspoon keto compliant Worcestershire sauce

- 2 teaspoons coconut aminos

Directions:

1. Season the roast with Italian seasoning, black pepper, garlic powder, and salt. Let it stand alone for about 27 to 30 minutes.

2. Add oil to a large skillet on medium-high heat. Add the roast; sear until brown, about 4 minutes on all sides.

3. Add the diced mushrooms and onions; let them cook for about 1 to 2 minutes until sweet-smelling.

4. Transfer the roast and the onions to the bottom of a slow cooker, then pour in the broth; then cook on high for 4 hours or low for 7 hours.

5. Add the vegetables: zucchini, celery, turnips, bell peppers, and cauliflower. Set it again for about 1 hour.

6. Transfer then shred into chunks with 2 forks.

7. Sprinkle with diced parsley if preferred. Serve hot with gravy.

Nutrition:

Calories: 345

Total Fat: 21g

Carbs: 4g

Fiber: 1g

Protein: 34g

CHAPTER 2:

Pork Recipes

8. Ginger & Lime Pork

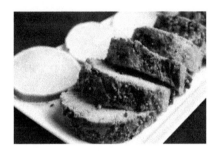

Preparation Time: 15 Minutes

Cooking Time: 8 Hours

Servings: 10

Ingredients:

- Salt and pepper to *taste*

- 1 tbsp. olive/avocado oil

- 1 t. stevia drops - vanilla

- 2 ½ lbs. pork loin

- 2 tbsp. low-carb brown sugar/molasses substitute

- 1/4 cup tamari

- 1 tbsp. Worcestershire sauce

- Juice of one lemon

- 1 tbsp. fresh ginger/½ t. ground

- ½ t. xanthan gum

- Optional: Fresh cilantro

Directions:

1. Prepare a large skillet on the stove top with the oil.

2. Rub the pepper and salt over the pork loin, and place it in hot oil in the skillet. Sear all sides until browned.

3. Take it from the burner, and place it in the bottom of the slow cooker.

4. Whisk together the ginger, garlic, lime juice, Worcestershire sauce, the sweeteners, and tamarin. Pour the mixture over the pork loin.

5. Place a cover on top of the slow cooker. Program the pork on high for four to seven hours or six hours on low. When finished arrange the pork on a platter and for the dishes in a small saucepan. sprinkle day xanthan gum on top. With the powder in

and cook until the mixture has thickened. Pour over the loin and garnish with some fresh cilantro.

Nutrition:

Calories: 292

Net Carbs: 1.9 g

Fat: 16 g

Protein: 31.9 g

9. Jamaican Jerk Pork Roast

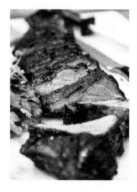

Preparation Time: 15 Minutes

Cooking Time: 4 Hours

Servings: 12

Ingredients:

- 1 (4 lb.) *pork shoulder*

- 1 tbsp. olive oil

- ½ c. Jamaican Jerk spice blend

- 1 c. beef broth/stock

Directions:

1. Coat the roast with olive oil and the Jerk spices.

2. Use a heavy-bottomed skillet to sear the meat.

3. Pour the cup of broth in the slow cooker, and arrange the meat in the bottom.

4. Cook for six hours on the low setting or four hours on the high setting.

Nutrition:

Calories: 282

Net Carbs: 0.0 g Fat: 20 g

Protein: 23 g

10. Pulled Pork

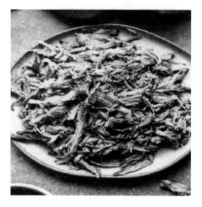

Preparation Time: 45 Minutes

Cooking Time: 6 Hours **Servings:** 8

Ingredients:

- 1 large white *onion*

- 3 bay leaves

- 3 ½ lb. pork shoulder

- 1/3 c. spicy chocolate barbecue sauce

Spices for Rub

- 1 tbsp. *of each:* Garlic powder, Paprika, Onion powder, and
  Smoked paprika

- ½ t. white or black pepper

Directions:

1. Set the temperature on your slow cooker to high.

2. Combine all of the spices in a mixing bowl. Use a sharp knife to score the skin of the pork approximately one-inch apart - going in both directions making it appear to have square cuts.

3. Rub the spices into the pork. Peel and crudely chop the onions, adding them to the slow cooker along with the bay leaves.

4. Arrange the pork on top and cover with the lid. Cook on low for 8 to 10 hours or high for five to six hours. It all depends on the size cooker you use.

5. When the pork is done, open the top and let the steam out. If you like a crispy top, preheat the oven temperature to 400°F.

6. Use two forks to transfer the pork onto the baking sheet that should be lined with parchment paper.

7. Use the barbecue sauce to cover the entire surface of the pork, and place it in the oven. Cook 30 to 40 minutes or until wanted brownness is accomplished.

8. Prepare the sauce. Combine the liquid with the cooked onions and bay leaves into a blender. Mix until smooth.

9. Remove the pork from the oven when done, and place it in a bowl.

10. Shred the meat bits, and pour the sauce from the blender over the top, and stir well.

11. Serve right away and enjoy with some roasted veggies.

Nutrition:

Calories: 497

Net Carbs: 3.8 g

Fat: 36.6 g

Protein: 35.0 g

CHAPTER 3:

Beef

11. Sweet Beef

Preparation time: 10 minutes **Cooking time:** 5 hours

Servings: 4 **Ingredients**

- 1-pound beef roast, sliced

- 1 tablespoon maple syrup

- 2 tablespoons lemon juice

- 1 teaspoon dried oregano

- 1 cup of water

Directions

1   Mix water with maple syrup, lemon juice, and dried oregano.

2   Then pour the liquid into the slow cooker.

3   Add beef roast and close the lid.

4   Cook the meal on High for 5 hours.

Nutrition: 227 calories, 34.5g protein, 3.8g carbohydrates, 7.2g fat, 0.2g fiber, 101mg cholesterol, 78mg sodium, 483mg potassium.

12. Thyme Beef

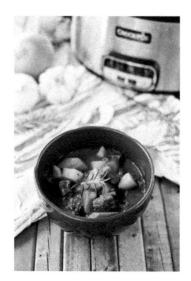

Preparation time: 15 minutes

Cooking time: 5 hours

Servings: 2

Ingredients

- 1/2 pound beef sirloin, chopped

- 1 tablespoon dried thyme

- 1 tablespoon olive oil

- ½ cup of water

- 1 teaspoon salt

Directions

1   Preheat the skillet well.

2   Then mix beef with dried thyme and olive oil.

3   Place the meat in the hot skillet and roast for 2 minutes per side on high heat.

4   Then transfer the meat to the slow cooker.

5   Add salt and water.

6   Cook the meal on High for 5 hours.

Nutrition :

274 calories, 34.5g protein

0.9g carbohydrates, 14.2g fat,

0.5g fiber 101mg cholesterol,

1240mg sodium, 469mg potassium

13. Hot Beef

Preparation time: 15 minutes

Cooking time: 8 hours

Servings: 4

Ingredients

- 1-pound beef sirloin, chopped

- 2 tablespoons hot sauce

- 1 tablespoon olive oil

- ½ cup of water

Directions

1   In the shallow bowl, mix hot sauce with olive oil.

2   Then mix beef sirloin with hot sauce mixture and leave for 10 minutes to marinate.

3   Put the marinated beef in the slow cooker.

4   Add water and close the lid.

5   Cook the meal on Low for 8 hours.

Nutrition :

241 calories, 34.4g protein, 0.1g carbohydrates, 10.6g fat, 0g fiber, 101mg cholesterol, 266mg sodium, 467mg potassium.

14. Beef Chops with Sprouts

Preparation time: 10 minutes **Cooking time:** 6 hours

Servings: 5 Ingredients

- 1-pound beef loin

- ½ cup bean sprouts

- 1 cup of water

- 1 tablespoon tomato paste

- 1 teaspoon chili powder

- 1 teaspoon salt

Directions

1   Cut the beef loin into 5 beef chops and sprinkle the beef chops

with chili powder and salt.

2   Then place them in the slow cooker.

3   Add water and tomato paste.

4   Cook the meat on low for 6 hours.

5   Then transfer the cooked beef chops onto the plates, sprinkle

with tomato gravy from the slow cooker, and top with bean sprouts.

Nutrition : 175 calories, 2 5.2g protein, 1.6g carbohydrates, 7.8g fat,

0.3g fiber, 64mg cholesterol, 526mg sodium, 386mg potassium.

15. Beef. Ragout with Beans

Preparation time: 10 minutes

Cooking time: 5 hours

Servings: 5

Ingredients

- 1 tablespoon tomato paste

- 1 cup mug beans, canned

- 1 carrot, grated

- 1-pound beef stew meat, chopped

- 1 teaspoon ground black pepper

- 2 cups of water

Directions

1   Pour water into the slow cooker.

2   Add meat, ground black pepper, and carrot.

3   Cook the mixture on High for 4 hours.

4   Then add tomato paste and mug beans. Stir the meal and cook it on high for 1 hour more.

Nutrition : 321 calories, 37.7g protein, 28g carbohydrates, 6.2g fat, 7.3g fiber, 81mg cholesterol, 81mg sodium, 959mg potassium.

16. Olives Beef. Stew

Preparation time: 10 minutes

Cooking time: 1o hours **Servings:** 4

Ingredients:

- 28 oz. beefsteak, cubed

- 1 tablespoon of olive oil

- 1 tablespoon of parsley, chopped

- Salt and black pepper- to taste

- 8 oz. tomato passata

- 1 yellow onion, diced

- 1 cup of green olives pitted

Directions:

1. Start by putting all the **Ingredients:** into your Slow cooker

2. Cover it and cook for 10 hours on Low settings.

3. Once done, uncover the pot and mix well.

4. Garnish as desired.

5. Serve warm. **Nutrition:** Calories 359 Total Fat 34 g Saturated Fat 10.3 g Cholesterol 112 mg Total Carbs 8.5 g Sugar 2 g Fiber 1.3 g Sodium 92 mg Protein 27.5 g

CHAPTER 4:

Lamb.

17. Lamb Leg with Thyme

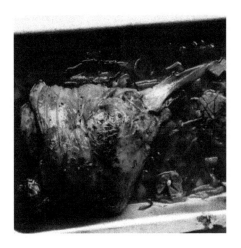

Preparation time: 10 minutes

Cooking time: 10 hours

Servings: 4

Ingredients

- 2 lbs. leg of lamb

- 1 teaspoon of fine salt

- 2 ½ tablespoons of olive oil

- 6 sprigs thyme

- 1 ½ cup of bone broth

- 6 garlic cloves, minced

- 1 ½ teaspoon of black pepper

- 1 ½ small onion

- 3/4 cup of vegetable stock

Directions:

1. Start by putting all the **Ingredients** into your Slow cooker.

2. Cover its lid and cook for 10 hours on Low settings.

3. Once done, remove its lid and mix well.

4. Garnish as desired.

5. Serve warm.

Nutrition:

Calories 112 Total Fat 4.9 g

Saturated Fat 1.9 g Cholesterol 10 mg

Sodium 355 mg

Total Carbs 1.9 g

Sugar 0.8 g

Fiber 0.4 g

Protein 3 g

18. Full Meal Turmeric Lamb

Preparation time: 10 minutes

Cooking time: 6 hours

Servings: 2

Ingredients

- ½ lb. ground lamb meat

- ½ cup of onion diced

- ½ tablespoon of garlic

- ½ tablespoon of minced ginger

- ¼ teaspoon of turmeric

- ¼ teaspoon of ground coriander

- ½ teaspoon of salt

- ¼ teaspoon of cumin

- ¼ teaspoon of cayenne pepper

Directions:

1. Start by putting all the **Ingredients** into your Slow cooker

2. Cover its lid and cook for 6 hours on Low settings.

3. Once done, remove its lid and mix well.

4. Garnish as desired.

5. Serve warm.

Nutrition:

Calories 132

Total Fat 10.9 g

Saturated Fat 2.7 g

Cholesterol 164 mg

Sodium 65 mg

Total Carbs 3.3 g

Sugar 0.5 g

Fiber 2.3 g

Protein 6.3 g

19. Lamb Cauliflower Curry

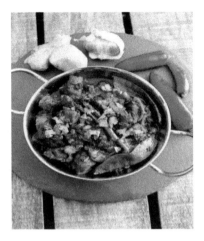

Preparation time: 10 minutes

Cooking time: 10 hours.

Servings: 4

Ingredients

- 2 lbs. lamb roasted Wegmans

- 1 cup of onion soup

- ¼ cup of carrots

- 1 cup of cauliflower

- 1 cup of beef broth

Directions:

1. Start by putting all the **Ingredients** into your Slow cooker

2. Cover its lid and cook for 10 hours on Low settings.

3. Once done, remove its lid and mix well.

4. Garnish as desired.

5. Serve warm.

Nutrition:

Calories 118 Total Fat 9.7 g Saturated Fat 4.3 g

Cholesterol 228 mg Sodium 160 mg Total Carbs 0.5 g Fiber 0 g Sugar

0.5 g Protein 7.4 g

CHAPTER 5:

Chicken

20. Green Chile Chicken

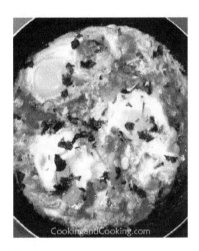

Preparation time: 10 minutes

Cooking time: 6 hours

Servings: 6

Ingredients:

- 8 chicken thighs, thawed, boneless and skinless

- 1 (4 oz.) can green chilis

- 2 teaspoons of garlic salt

- optional: add in ½ cup of diced onions

Directions:

1. Start by throwing all the Ingredients into the Slow cooker

2. Cover it and cook for 6 hours on Low Settings.

3. Garnish as desired.

4. Serve warm.

Nutrition:

Calories 248 Total Fat 2.4 g

Saturated Fat 0.1 g

Cholesterol 320 mg

Total Carbs 2.9 g

Fiber 0.7 g Sugar 0.7 g

Sodium 350 mg

Potassium 255 mg

Protein 44.3 g

21. Garlic Butter Chicken with Cream Cheese Sauce

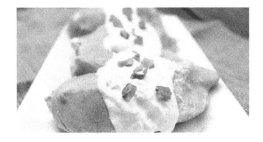

Preparation time: 10 minutes

Cooking time: 6 hours

Servings: 4

Ingredients:

For the garlic chicken:

- 8 garlic cloves, sliced

- 1.5 teaspoons of salt

- 1 stick of butter

- 2 2.5 lbs. of chicken breasts

- Optional 1 onion, sliced

For the cream cheese sauce:

- 8 oz. of cream cheese

- 1 cup of chicken stock

- salt to taste

Directions:

1. Start by throwing all the Ingredients for garlic chicken into the Slow cooker

2. Cover it and cook for 6 hours on Low Settings.

3. Now stir cook all the Ingredients for cream cheese sauce in a saucepan.

4. Once heated, pour this sauce over the cooked chicken.

5. Garnish as desired.

6. Serve warm.

Nutrition:

- Calories 301

Total Fat 12.2 g

Saturated Fat 2.4 g

Cholesterol 110 mg

Total Carbs 1.5 g

Fiber 0.9 g

Sugar 1.4 g

Sodium 276 mg

Potassium 375mg

Protein 28.8 g

22. Jerk chicken

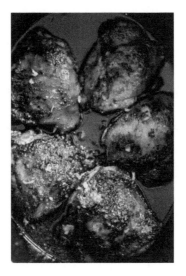

Preparation time: 10 minutes

Cooking time: 6 hours

Servings: 5

Ingredients

- 5 drumsticks and 5 wings

- 4 teaspoons of salt

- 4 teaspoons of paprika

- 1 teaspoon of cayenne pepper

- 2 teaspoons of onion powder

- 2 teaspoons of thyme

- 2 teaspoons of white pepper

- 2 teaspoons of garlic powder

- 1 teaspoon of black pepper

Directions:

1. Start by throwing all the Ingredients into the Slow cooker

2. Cover it and cook for 6 hours on Low Settings.

3. Garnish as desired.

4. Serve warm.

Nutrition:

Calories 249

Total Fat 11.9 g

Saturated Fat 1.7 g

Cholesterol 78 mg

Total Carbs 1.8 g

Fiber 1.1 g Sugar 0.3 g

Sodium 79 mg

Potassium 264 mg

Protein 35 g

23. Spicy Wings with Mint Sauce

Preparation time: 10 minutes

Cooking time: 6 hours

Servings: 6

Ingredients

- 1 tablespoon of cumin

- 18 chicken wings, cut in half

- 1 tablespoon of turmeric

- 1 tablespoon of coriander

- 1 tablespoon of fresh ginger, finely grated

- 2 tablespoon of olive oil

- 1 tablespoon of paprika

- A pinch of cayenne pepper

- ¼ cup of chicken stock

- Salt and black pepper ground, to taste

Chutney/ Sauce:

- 1 cup of fresh mint leaves

- Juice of ½ lime

- ¾ cup of cilantro

- 1 Serrano pepper

- 1 tablespoon of water

- 1 small ginger piece, peeled and diced

- 1 tablespoon of olive oil

- Salt and black pepper ground, to taste

Directions:

1. Start by throwing all the **Ingredients** for wings into the Slow cooker

2. Cover it and cook for 6 hours on Low Settings.

3. Meanwhile, blend all the mint sauce **Ingredients** in a blender jug.

4. Serve the cooked wings with mint sauce.

5. Garnish as desired.

6. Serve warm.

Nutrition: Calories 248 Total Fat 15.7 g Saturated Fat 2.7 g Cholesterol 75 mg Total Carbs 0.4 g Fiber 0g Sugar 0 g Sodium 94 mg Potassium 158 mg Protein 24.9 g

24. Cacciatore Olive Chicken

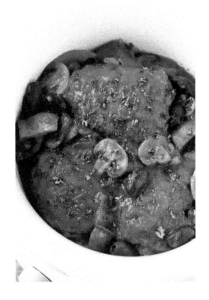

Preparation time: 10 minutes

Cooking time: 6 hours

Servings: 4

Ingredients

- 28 oz. canned tomatoes and juice, crushed

- 8 chicken drumsticks, bone-in

- 1 cup of chicken stock

- 1 bay leaf

- 1 teaspoon of garlic powder

- 1 yellow onion, diced

- 1 teaspoon of oregano, dried

- salt to taste

Directions:

1. Start by throwing all the **Ingredients** into the Slow cooke and mix them well.

2. Cover it and cook for 6 hours on Low Settings.

3. Garnish as desired.

4. Serve warm.

Nutrition:

Calories 297 Total Fat 16.2 g Saturated Fat 6.5 g

Cholesterol 35 mg Total Carbs 5.9 g Sugar 3.3 g

Fiber 1.9 g Sodium 575 mg Potassium 155 mg

Protein 8.9 g

25. Duck and Vegetable Stew

Preparation time: 10 minutes **Cooking time:** 5 hours

Servings: 4

Ingredients

- 1 duck, diced into medium pieces

- 1 tablespoon of wine

- 2 carrots, diced

- 2 cups of water

- 1 cucumber, diced

- 1-inch ginger pieces, diced

- Salt and black pepper- to taste

Directions:

1. Start by throwing all the **Ingredients** except into the Slow cooker and mix them well.

2. Cover it and cook for 5 hours on Low Settings.

3. Garnish with cucumber.

Nutrition: Calories 449 Total Fat 23.4 g Saturated Fat 1.5 g Cholesterol 210 mg Total Carbs 0.4 g Fiber 1.3 g Sugar 22g Sodium 838 mg Potassium 331 mg Protein 28.5g

CHAPTER 6:

Seafood

26. Spicy Barbecue Shrimp

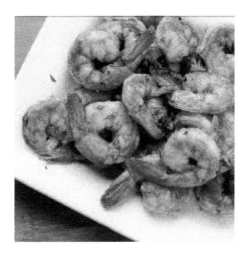

Preparation Time: 5 Minutes

Cooking Time: 1 Hour and 30 Minutes

Servings: 6

Ingredients:

- 1 1/2 pounds large wild-caught shrimp, unpeeled

- 1 green onion, chopped

- 1 teaspoon minced garlic

- 1 ½ teaspoon salt

- ¾ teaspoon ground black pepper

- 1 teaspoon Cajun seasoning

- 1 tablespoon hot pepper sauce

- ¼ cup Worcestershire Sauce

- 1 lemon, juiced

- 2 tablespoons avocado oil

- 1/2 cup unsalted butter, chopped

Directions:

1. Place all the ingredients except for shrimps in a 6-quart slow cooker and whisk until mixed.

2. Plug in the slow cooker, then shut with lid and cook for 30 minutes at high heat setting.

3. Then take out ½ cup of this sauce and reserve.

4. Add shrimps to slow cooker.

Nutrition:

Net Carbs: 2.4g; Calories: 321; Total Fat: 21.4g; Saturated Fat: 10.6g;

Protein: 27.3g; Carbs: 4.8g;

Fiber: 2.4g;

Sugar: 1.2g

27. Lemon Dill Halibut

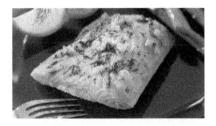

Preparation Time: 5 Minutes

Cooking Time: 2 Hours **Servings:** 2 **Ingredients:**

- 12-ounce wild-caught halibut fillet

- 1 teaspoon salt

- ½ teaspoon ground black pepper

- 1 1/2 teaspoon dried dill

- 1 tablespoon fresh lemon juice

- 3 tablespoons avocado oil

Directions:

1. Cut an 18-inch piece of aluminum foil, place halibut fillet in the middle and then season with salt and black pepper.

2. Whisk together remaining ingredients, drizzle this mixture over halibut, then crimp the edges of foil and place it into a 6-quart slow cooker.

3. Plug in the slow cooker, shut with lid and cook for 1 hour and 30 minutes or 2 hours at high heat setting or until cooked through.

4. When done, carefully open the crimped edges and check the fish, it should be tender and flaky. Serve straightaway.

Nutrition:

Net Carbs: 0g; Calories: 321.5; Total Fat: 21.4g; Saturated Fat: 7.2g; Protein: 32.1g; Carbs: 0g; Fiber: 0g; Sugar: 0.6g

28. Coconut Cilantro Curry Shrimp

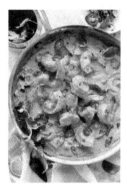

Preparation Time: 5 Minutes

Cooking Time: 2 Hours and 30 Minutes

Servings: 4

Ingredients:

- 1 pound wild-caught shrimp, peeled and deveined

- 2 ½ teaspoon lemon garlic seasoning

- 2 tablespoons red curry paste

- 4 tablespoons chopped cilantro

- 30 ounces coconut milk, unsweetened

- 16 ounces water

Directions:

1. Whisk together all the ingredients except for shrimps and 2 tablespoons cilantro and add to a 4-quart slow cooker.

2. Plug in the slow cooker, shut with lid and cook for 2 hours at high heat setting or 4 hours at low heat setting.

3. Then add shrimps, toss until evenly coated and cook for 20 to 30 minutes at high heat settings or until shrimps are pink.

4. Garnish shrimps with remaining cilantro and serve.

Nutrition: Net Carbs: 1.9g; Calories: 160.7; Total Fat: 8.2g; Saturated Fat: 8.1g; Protein: 19.3g; Carbs: 2.4g; Fiber: 0.5g; Sugar: 1.4g

CHAPTER 7:

Vegetables

29. Slow cooker Parmesan Lemon Cauliflower

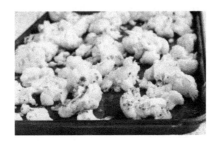

Preparation time: 15 minutes

Cooking time: 2 hours

Servings: 4

Ingredients:

- 1-pound cauliflower

- 2 tablespoons butter

- 2 tablespoons fresh sage or powdered

- 2 tablespoons lemon juice

- 1 cup parmesan cheese

- Parsley to garnish

Directions:

1. Place all the fixing in a bowl and thoroughly cover the cauliflower with the butter, sage, and lemon. Cook on low for 2 hours.

2. Once done, add parmesan cheese and a bit more lemon and let it steam for 10 minutes. Serve with a topping of fresh parsley.

Nutrition:

Calories: 180Fat: 18g

Protein: 3g

Carbs: 18g

30. Garlic Herb Mushrooms

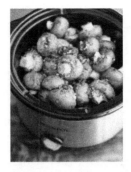

Preparation time: 15 minutes

Cooking time: 4 hours Servings: 4Ingredients:

- ¼ teaspoon thyme

- 2 bay leaves - 1 cup vegetable broth

- ½ cup half and half

- 2 tablespoons butter

- 2 tablespoons fresh parsley, chopped

- Salt and pepper, to taste

Directions:

Place all of the ingredients save for the butter and the half and half in the slow cooker and put on low for 3 hours. Once done, add the butter and half and half for the last 15 minutes. Garnish with parsley and enjoy.

Nutrition: Calories: 175 Fat: 18g Protein: 3g Carbs: 18g

31. Sticky Sesame Cauliflower Slow Cooker Bites

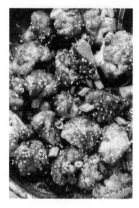

Preparation time: 15 minutes

Cooking time: 2 hours Servings: 4

Ingredients:

- 1-pound cauliflower - ½ teaspoon paprika - ½ teaspoon ground cumin

- 1 teaspoon garlic powder

- 1 teaspoon sesame oil

- 1/3 cup honey

- 2 tablespoons apple cider vinegar

- 1 teaspoon sweet chili sauce

- 3 garlic cloves, minced

- ¼ cup of water

- 1 tablespoon arrowroot powder or cornstarch

- 1 cup green onions to garnish

- Sesame seeds to garnish

Directions:

1. Place all spices, minus the green onions and sesame seeds, in a bowl, and cover the cauliflower thoroughly with the mixture. Place the cauliflower into the slow cooker.

2. Add the rest of the ingredients and cover. Cook on low for 2 hours. The sauce will thicken with the cornstarch or arrowroot powder. When done, remove each bite and garnish with toasted sesame seeds and green onion slices on top.

Nutrition: Calories: 240 Fat: 7g Protein: 3g Carbs: 18g

32. Slow cooker Cauliflower Mac and Cheese

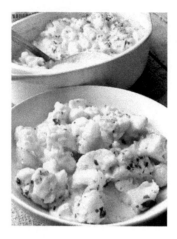

Preparation time: 15 minutes

Cooking time: 4 hours Servings: 4

Ingredients:

- 1-pound cauliflower

- 2 cups shredded cheddar cheese

- 2 ½ cups milk

- 1 12-ounce can evaporate milk

- ½ tablespoon mustard

Directions:

1. Place all of the fixings above in the slow cooker and put on low

   for 3 hours until most of the liquid has been absorbed.

2. Sprinkle some extra cheese on top and cook for 15 minutes until it has melted and the rest of the liquid is absorbed. Garnish with some parsley and even shredded parmesan cheese.

Nutrition: Calories: 215 Fat: 4g Protein: 3g Carbs: 18g

CHAPTER 8:

Desserts

33. Pumpkin Spice Pudding

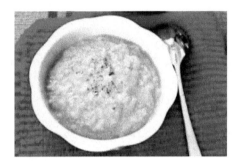

Preparation Time: 5 Minutes

Cooking Time: 8 Hours **Servings:** 10

Ingredients:

- 3 tablespoons melted coconut oil

- 2 cups canned coconut milk

- 1½ cups puréed pumpkin

- 4 large eggs, lightly beaten

- 1 tablespoon pure vanilla extract

- ½ cup erythritol

- ¼ cup almond flour

- 2 teaspoons pumpkin pie spice

- 1 teaspoon stevia powder

- 1 teaspoon baking powder

Directions:

1. Coat the inside of your slow cooker insert with coconut oil.

2. In the insert, stir together 3 tablespoons of coconut oil, coconut milk, pumpkin, eggs, vanilla, erythritol, almond flour, pumpkin pie spice, stevia powder, and baking powder until smooth. Cover then cook it for 8 hours on low.

3. Serve warm or you may refrigerate it for up to 3 days and serve chilled.

Nutrition: Calories: 215 Total fat: 19g Protein: 4g

Total carbs: 7g Fiber: 3g

Net carbs: 4g Sodium: 34mg

Cholesterol: 65mg

34. Chocolate & Coconut Pudding

Preparation Time: 10 Minutes

Cooking Time: 8 Hours

Servings: 10

Ingredients:

- 3 tablespoons melted coconut oil, plus more for coating the slow cooker insert
- 4 ounces unsweetened chocolate, chopped
- 2 cups canned coconut milk
- 4 large eggs, lightly beaten
- 2 teaspoons coconut extract
- 1 teaspoon pure vanilla extract
- ½ cup erythritol
- ¼ cup almond flour
- 1 teaspoon stevia powder
- 1 teaspoon baking powder

Directions:

1. Coat the inside of the slow cooker with coconut oil.

2. In a microwave-safe bowl or measuring cup, combine 3 tablespoons of coconut oil with the chocolate. Microwave for 1 minute on high. Stir, and then microwave in 30-second intervals, stirring in between, until the chocolate is melted and smooth. Transfer to the prepared insert.

3. Stir in the coconut milk, eggs, coconut and vanilla extracts, erythritol, almond flour, stevia powder, and baking powder until smooth. Cover then cook it for 8 hours on low. Serve it warm or you may refrigerate it for up to 3 days and serve chilled.

Nutrition:

Calories: 223

Total fat: 19g

Protein: 5g

Total carbs: 8g

Fiber: 3g

Net carbs: 5g

Sodium: 35mg

Cholesterol: 65mg

35. Coconut-Raspberry Cake

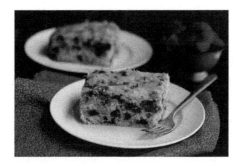

Preparation Time: 10 Minutes

Cooking Time: 3 Hours **Servings:** 10

Ingredients:

- ½ cup melted coconut oil

- 2 cups almond flour

- 1 cup unsweetened shredded coconut

- 1 cup erythritol or 1 teaspoon stevia powder

- ¼ cup unsweetened, unflavored protein powder

- 2 teaspoons baking soda

- ¼ teaspoon fine sea salt

- 4 large eggs, lightly beaten

- ¾ cup canned coconut milk

- 1 teaspoon coconut extract

- 1 cup raspberries, fresh or frozen

Directions:

1. Coat the inside of the slow cooker with coconut oil.

2. In a bowl, stir the almond flour, coconut, erythritol, protein powder, baking soda, and sea salt.

3. Whisk in the eggs, coconut milk, ½ cup of coconut oil, and coconut extract.

4. Gently fold in the raspberries.

5. Move the batter to the prepared slow cooker, cover, and cook for 3 hours on low. Turn off the slow cooker then allow the cake cool for several hours, to room temperature. Serve at room temperature.

Nutrition: Calories: 405 Total fat: 38g Protein: 11g Total carbs: 10g Fiber: 5g Net carbs: 5g Sodium: 358mg Cholesterol: 127mg

36. Tangy Lemon Cake with Lemon Glaze

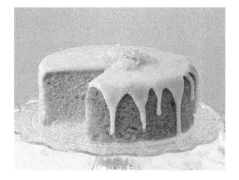

Preparation Time: 10 Minutes

Cooking Time: 3 or 6 Hours **Servings:** 8

Ingredients:

FOR THE GLAZE

- ½ cup boiling water

- ¼ cup erythritol

- 2 tablespoons unsalted butter or Ghee, melted

- 2 tablespoons freshly squeezed lemon juice

FOR THE CAKE

- Coconut oil, for coating the insert

- 2 cups almond flour

- ½ cup erythritol

- 2 teaspoons baking powder

- 3 large eggs

- ½ cup (1 stick) unsalted butter, melted and cooled slightly

- ½ cup heavy (whipping) cream

- Grated zest and juice of 2 lemons

Directions:

TO MAKE THE GLAZE

1. In a small bowl, stir together all the ingredients. Set aside.

TO MAKE THE CAKE

2. Coat the inside of the slow cooker also put the coconut oil.

3. In a medium bowl, blend the almond flour, erythritol, and baking powder.

4. In a bowl, beat the eggs, then whisk in the butter, heavy cream, lemon zest, and lemon juice.

5. Add the dry fixings to the wet fixings. Stir to mix well. Transfer the batter to the insert and spread evenly with a rubber spatula.

6. Pour the glaze over the cake batter. Cover then cook it for 6 hours on low or 3 hours on high. Serve warm or at room temperature.

Nutrition: Calories: 420 Total fat: 40g Protein: 11g Total carbs: 10g Fiber: 4g Net carbs: 6g Sodium: 45mg Cholesterol: 137mg

37. Moist Ginger Cake with Whipped Cream

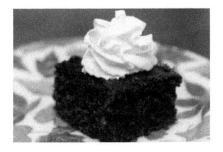

Preparation Time: 15 Minutes

Cooking Time: 3 Hours **Servings:** 10

Ingredients:

FOR THE CAKE

- ½ cup (1 stick) unsalted butter, melted

- 2¼ cups almond flour

- ¾ cup erythritol

- 2 tablespoons coconut flour

- 1½ tablespoons ground ginger

- 1 tablespoon unsweetened cocoa powder

- 2 teaspoons baking powder

- 1½ teaspoons ground cinnamon

- ½ teaspoon ground cloves

- ¼ teaspoon fine sea salt

- 4 large eggs, lightly beaten

- 2/3 cup heavy (whipping) cream

- 1 teaspoon pure vanilla extract

FOR THE WHIPPED CREAM

- 1 cup heavy (whipping) cream

- ½ teaspoon stevia powder or ½ cup erythritol- 1 teaspoon pure vanilla extract

Directions:

TO MAKE THE CAKE

1. Coat the inside of the slow cooker insert with butter.

2. In a large bowl, mix the almond flour, erythritol, coconut flour, ginger, cocoa powder, baking powder, cinnamon, cloves, and sea salt.

3. Add butter, eggs, heavy cream, and vanilla. Mix and transfer to the insert.

4. Cover and cook for 3 hours on low. Serve warm with whipped cream.

TO MAKE THE WHIPPED CREAM

5. In a large bowl, with the use of an electric mixer set on medium-high to beat the heavy cream, stevia, and vanilla until stiff peaks form, about 5 minutes.

Nutrition:

Calories: 453 Total fat: 43g Protein: 12g Total carbs: 12g Fiber: 5g Net carbs: 7g Sodium: 103mg Cholesterol: 109mg

38. Chocolate–Macadamia Nut Cheesecake

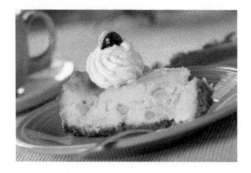

Preparation Time: 15 Minutes

Cooking Time: 2 or 4 Hours **Servings:** 8

Ingredients:

FOR THE CRUST

- 1 cup macadamia nuts, ground to a meal

- 1 large egg, lightly beaten

- 2 tablespoons coconut oil, melted

- 1 teaspoon stevia powder

- 1 cup water

FOR THE FILLING

- 6 ounces unsweetened chocolate, chopped

- 2 large eggs

- 2 (8-ounce) packages cream cheese

- ¼ cup coconut cream

- 1 tablespoon coconut flour

- 1 teaspoon pure vanilla extract

- ½ cup erythritol

- ½ teaspoon stevia powder

- ¼ cup coarsely chopped macadamia nuts

Directions:

TO MAKE THE CRUST

1. In a medium bowl, stir together the macadamia nut meal, egg, coconut oil, and stevia powder. Press the combination into the bottom of a baking pan that fits into your slow cooker (make sure there is room on the sides so you can lift the pan out). An oval baking dish, round cake pan, or loaf pan could all work, depending on the size and shape of your slow cooker.

2. Pour the water into the slow cooker insert. Place the pan in the cooker.

TO MAKE THE FILLING

1. In a microwave-safe bowl, heat the chocolate in the microwave for 1 minute on high. Stir and then microwave in 30-second

intervals, stirring in between, until the chocolate is melted and smooth. Set it aside.

2. In a large bowl, beat the eggs, then beat in the cream cheese, coconut cream, coconut flour, vanilla, erythritol, and stevia powder.

3. Stir in the chocolate until well incorporated. Pour the mixture over the crust. Cover then cook it for 4 hours on low or 2 hours on high.

4. When done, turn off the slow cooker and let the cheesecake sit inside until cooled to room temperature, up to 3 hours.

5. Remove the pan from the slow cooker and refrigerate until chilled, about 2 hours more.

6. Sprinkle the macadamia nuts over the top and serve chilled.

Nutrition: Calories: 433 Total fat: 44g Protein: 8g

Total carbs: 6g Fiber: 2g Net carbs: 4g Sodium: 208mg Cholesterol: 141mg

39. Vanilla Cheesecake

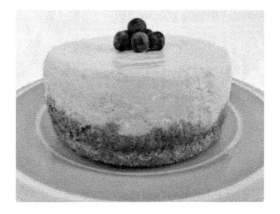

Preparation Time: 15 Minutes

Cooking Time: 2 or 4 Hours

Servings: 8

Ingredients:

FOR THE CRUST

- 1 cup toasted walnuts, ground to a meal

- 1 large egg, lightly beaten

- 2 tablespoons coconut oil, melted

- 1 teaspoon stevia powder

- 1 cup water

FOR THE FILLING

- 2 large eggs

- 2 (8-ounce) packages cream cheese

- ¼ cup heavy (whipping) cream

- 2 teaspoons pure vanilla extract

- ½ cup erythritol

- 1 tablespoon coconut flour

- ½ teaspoon stevia powder

Directions:

TO MAKE THE CRUST

1. In a medium bowl, blend the walnut meal, egg, coconut oil, and stevia powder. Press the mixture into the bottom part of a baking pan that fits into your slow cooker (make sure there is room to lift the pan out). An oval baking dish, round cake pan, or loaf pan could all work, depending on the size and shape of your slow cooker.

2. Pour the water into the slow cooker insert. Place the pan in the cooker.

TO MAKE THE FILLING

3. In a large bowl, beat the eggs and the cream cheese, heavy cream, vanilla, erythritol, coconut flour, and stevia powder. Pour

the mixture over the crust. Cover then cook it for 4 hours on low or 2 hours on high.

4. When finished, turn off the cooker and let the cheesecake sit inside until cooled to room temperature, up to 3 hours.

5. Remove the pan from the slow cooker and refrigerate until chilled, about 2 hours more. Serve chilled.

Nutrition: Calories: 338 Total fat: 33g Protein: 7g Total carbs: 5g Fiber: 1g Net carbs: 4g Sodium: 208mg Cholesterol: 146mg

40. Toasted Almond Cheesecake

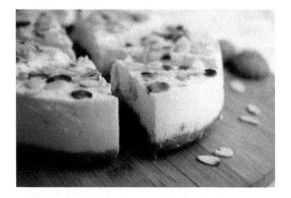

Preparation Time: 15 Minutes

Cooking Time: 2 or 4 Hours **Servings:** 8

Ingredients:

FOR THE CRUST

- 1 cup toasted almonds, ground to a meal

- 1 large egg, lightly beaten

- 2 tablespoons coconut oil, melted

- 1 teaspoon stevia powder

- 1 cup water

FOR THE FILLING

- 2 large eggs

- 2 (8-ounce) packages cream cheese

- ¾ cup almond butter

- ¼ cup coconut cream

- 1 teaspoon pure almond extract

- ¾ cup erythritol

- 1 tablespoon coconut flour

- 2 teaspoons stevia powder

Directions:

TO MAKE THE CRUST

1. In a medium bowl, mix the almond meal, egg, coconut oil, and stevia powder. Press the mixture into the bottom part of a baking pan that fits into your slow cooker (make sure there is room to lift the pan out). Many pans could work, depending on the size and shape of your slow cooker.

2. Pour the water into the slow cooker insert. Place the pan in the cooker.

TO MAKE THE FILLING

3. In a large bowl, beat the eggs and the cream cheese, almond butter, coconut cream, almond extract, erythritol, coconut flour, and stevia powder. Pour the mixture over the crust. Cover then cook it for 4 hours on low or 2 hours on high.

4. When done, turn off the slow cooker and let the cheesecake sit inside until cooled to room temperature, up to 3 hours.

5. Take away the pan from the slow cooker and refrigerate until chilled, about 2 hours more. Serve chilled.

Nutrition:

Calories: 538

Total fat: 51g

Protein: 14g

Total carbs: 12g

Fiber: 3g

Net carbs: 9g

Sodium: 215mg

Cholesterol: 141mg

CHAPTER 9:

Soups

41. German Style Soup

Preparation time: 15 minutes

Cooking time: 8.5 Hours

Servings: 6

Ingredients

- 1-pound beef loin, chopped

- 6 cups of water

- 1 cup sauerkraut

- 1 onion, diced

- 1 teaspoon cayenne pepper

- ½ cup Greek yogurt

Directions:

1. Put beef and onion in the Slow Cooker

2. Add yogurt, water, and cayenne pepper.

3. Cook the mixture on low for 8 hours.

4. When the beef is cooked, add sauerkraut and stir the soup carefully.

5. Cook the soup on high for 30 minutes.

Nutrition:

137 calories, 16.1g protein, 4.3g carbohydrates,

 5.8g fat, 1.1g fiber, 41mg cholesterol,

503mg sodium,

93mg potassium.

42. Shrimp Chowder

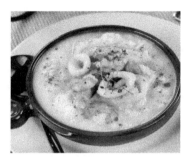

Preparation time: 15 minutes**Cooking time:** 1 Hour **Servings:** 4

Ingredients

- 1-pound shrimps

- ½ cup fennel bulb, chopped

- 1 bay leaf

- ½ teaspoon peppercorn

- 1 cup of coconut milk

- 3 cups of water

- 1 teaspoon ground coriander

Directions:

1. Put all **Ingredients:** in the Slow Cooker

2. Close the lid and cook the chowder on High for 1 hour.

Nutrition: 277 calories, 27.4g protein, 6.1g carbohydrates, 16.3g fat, 1.8g fiber, 239mg cholesterol, 297mg sodium, 401mg potassium.

43. Ground Pork. Soup

Preparation time: 15 minutes

Cooking time: 5.5 Hour **Servings:** 4

Ingredients

- 1 cup ground pork

- ½ cup red kidney beans, canned

- 1 cup tomatoes, canned

- 4 cups of water

- 1 tablespoon dried cilantro

- 1 teaspoon salt

Directions:

1. Put ground pork in the Slow Cooker

2. Add tomatoes, water, dried cilantro, and salt. Close the lid and cook the **Ingredients:** on High for 5 hours.

3. Then add canned red kidney beans and cook the soup on high for 30 minutes more.

Nutrition: 318 calories, 25.7g protein, 10.9g carbohydrates, 16.6g fat, 4.1g fiber, 74mg cholesterol, 651mg sodium, 706mg potassium.

44. Chinese Style Cod

Preparation time: 15 minutes

Cooking time: 5 Hours **Servings:** 2

Ingredients

- 6 oz. cod fillet

- 1 teaspoon sesame seeds

- 1 teaspoon olive oil

- 1 garlic clove, chopped

- ¼ cup of soy sauce

- ¼ cup fish stock

- 4 oz. fennel bulb, chopped

Directions:

1. Pour fish stock in the Slow Cooker

2. Add soy sauce, olive oil, garlic, and sesame seeds.

3. Then chop the fish roughly and add in the Slow Cooker

4. Cook the meal on Low for 5 hours.

Nutrition: 139 calories, 18.9g protein, 7.4g carbohydrates, 4.2g fat, 2.2g fiber, 42mg cholesterol, 1926mg sodium, 359mg potassium.

45. Beans. Stew.

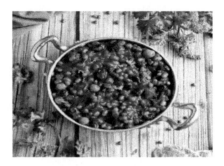

Preparation time: 15 minutes

Cooking time: 5 Hours **Servings:** 3

Ingredients

- ½ cup sweet pepper, chopped

- ¼ cup onion, chopped

- 1 cup edamame beans

- 1 cup tomatoes

- 1 teaspoon cayenne pepper

- 5 cups of water

- 2 tablespoons cream cheese

Directions:

1. Mix water with cream cheese and pour the liquid in the Slow
   Cooker

2. Add cayenne pepper, edamame beans, and onion.

3. Then chop the tomatoes roughly and add in the Slow Cooker

4. Close the lid and cook the stew on high for 5 hurs.

Nutrition: 74 calories, 3.4g protein, 7.9g carbohydrates, 3.6g fat, 2.4g

fiber, 7mg cholesterol, 109mg sodium,

218mg potassium.

46. Creamy Bacon Soupr

Preparation time: 15 minutes

Cooking time: 1 3/4 Hours

Servings: 6

Ingredients

- 1 tablespoon olive oil

- 6 bacon slices, chopped

- 1 sweet onion, chopped

- 1 1/2 pounds' potatoes, peeled and cubed

- 1 parsnip, diced

- 1/2 celery root, cubed

- 2 cups chicken stock

- 3 cups water

- Salt and pepper to taste

Directions:

1. Heat the oil in a skillet and add the bacon. Cook until crisp then remove the bacon on a plate.

2. Pour the fat of the bacon in your Slow Cooker and add the remaining Ingredients.

3. Adjust the taste with salt and pepper and cook on high settings for 1 1/2 hours.

4. When done, puree the soup with an immersion blender until smooth.

5. Pour the soup in a bowl and top with bacon.

6. Serve right away.

Nutrition:

calories 187, fat 4, fiber 4, carbs 7,

protein 8

47. Seafood Stew

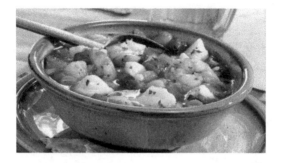

Preparation time: 15 minutes

Cooking time: 7 Hours

Servings: 4

Ingredients

- 28 ounces canned tomatoes, crushed

- 4 cups veggie stock

- 3 garlic cloves, minced

- 1 pound sweet potatoes, cubed

- ½ cup yellow onion, chopped

- 2 pounds mixed seafood

- 1 teaspoon thyme, dried

- 1 teaspoon cilantro, dried

- 1 teaspoon basil, dried

- Salt and black pepper to the taste

- A pinch of red pepper flakes, crushed

Directions:

1. In your Slow Cooker, mix tomatoes with stock, garlic, sweet potatoes, onion, thyme, cilantro, basil, salt, pepper and pepper flakes, stir, cover and cook on Low 6 hours.

2. Add seafood, stir, cover, and cook on High for 1 more hours, divide stew into bowls, and serve lunch.

Nutrition:

calories 270,

fat 4,

fiber 4,

carbs 12,

protein 3

48. Swedish Pea and Ham Soup

Preparation Time: 10 Minutes

Cooking Time: 5 Hours

Servings: 8

Ingredients:

- 3 cups yellow split peas, rinsed and drained

- 4 cups water

- 4 cups low sodium chicken stock

- 1 cup carrots, diced

- 2 cups onions, diced

- 1 tbsp. fresh ginger, minced

- 8 oz. ham, sliced

- 1 tsp. dried marjoram

- 1/4 tsp. pepper

Directions:

1. Put the split peas, water, stock, carrots, onions, celery, ginger, ham, and marjoram in the slow cooker.

2. Stir to blend everything. Put the lid on.

3. For 4 hours and 30 minutes to 5 hours, cook it on high.

4. Season with pepper before serving. Enjoy!

Nutrition:

Calories 338,

Fat 3,

Carbs 23,

Protein 21

49. Fisherman's Stew

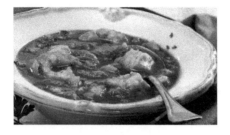

Preparation Time: 17 Minutes

Cooking Time: 8 Hours and 35 Minutes

Servings: 6

Ingredients:

- 2 tbsp. olive oil

- 2 garlic cloves, finely chopped

- 1 cup baby carrots, sliced 1/4 inch thick

- 6 large Roma tomatoes, sliced and quartered

- 1 green bell pepper, chopped

- 1/2 tsp. fennel seed

- 1 cup water

- 1 bottle (8 oz.) clam juice

- 1-pound cod, cut into 1-inch cubes

- 1/2-pound medium shrimp, uncooked, peeled, and deveined

- 1 tsp. stevia

- 1 tsp. dried basil leaves

- 1/2 tsp. salt

- 1/4 tsp. red pepper sauce

- 2 tbsp. fresh parsley, chopped

Directions:

1. Stir the olive oil, garlic, carrots, tomatoes, green pepper, fennel seed, water, and clam juice together in the slow cooker.

2. Cover then cook it for 8 to 9 hours on LOW. Vegetables should be tender.

3. Twenty minutes before serving, add cod, shrimp, stevia, basil, salt, and pepper sauce.

4. Cover and cook 15 to 20 minutes on HIGH. The soup is ready when the fish can easily be flaked and shrimp are pink in color. Serve and enjoy!

Nutrition:

Calories 180,

Fat 26, Carbs 10, Protein 10

50. Seafood Gumbo

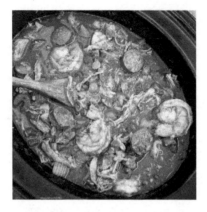

Preparation Time: 17 Minutes

Cooking Time: 2 Hours and 20 Minutes **Servings:** 6

Ingredients:

- 8 to 10 bacon strips, sliced

- 2 stalks celery, sliced

- 1 medium onion, sliced

- 1 green pepper, chopped

- 2 garlic cloves, minced

- 2 cups chicken broth

- 1 can (14 oz.) diced tomatoes, undrained

- 2 tbsp. Worcestershire sauce

- 2 tsp. salt

- 1 tsp. dried thyme leaves

- 1-pound large raw shrimp, peeled, deveined

- 1 pound fresh or frozen crabmeat

- 1 box (10 oz.) frozen okra, thawed and sliced into 1/2-inch pieces

Directions:

1. Brown the bacon in a skillet through medium heat. When crisp, drain and transfer to a slow cooker.

2. Drain off drippings, leaving just enough to coat the skillet.

3. Sauté celery, onion, green pepper, and garlic until vegetables are tender.

4. Transfer the sautéed vegetables to the slow cooker.

5. Add the broth, tomatoes, Worcestershire sauce, salt, and thyme.

6. Cover then cook it for 4 hours on LOW, or for 2 hours on HIGH.

7. Add the shrimp, crabmeat, and okra. Cover and cook 1 hour longer on LOW or 30 minutes longer on HIGH. Serve and enjoy!

Nutrition: Calories 263, Fat 8, Carbs 13, Protein 4

Conclusion

As you go along, as you now know so many new ways to cook your food, just decide which one you want to make first for your family and friends. Make a list of all the ingredients needed to prepare the different meals. Each of the provided recipes has provided the nutritional factors you need to prepare a healthy meal. You will learn how easy it is to prepare these meals. It will be much easier to calculate the carbohydrates you eat daily.

Here are some tips to keep you on track when on the ketogenic diet:

- Reheat tasty leftovers.
- Eat low-carb snacks.
- Drink coffee or tea instead of something sweet.

Anyone can make mistakes. Here are a few to keep in mind when using your keto recipes to get healthier:

- Maintain discipline. All you have to do is stay determined with your goals by moving from regular to ketogenic meals.
- Listen to your body. Your body knows more than you think because it understands how many servings of food you need to maintain your exercise routine. If you are hungry, eat; if you are not hungry, do not eat.
- Don't look for shortcuts. Try to plan your meals so as not to eat carbohydrates that are wasted on junk food. Save carbohydrates for food as a special treat. Resist the urge to eat that bag of chips. Instead, why not eat some tasty fruit?
- Do not go out. It will take more than a few days to get your plan in place. Follow the guidelines provided in this book because they are calculated based on the carbohydrates, fats, and proteins your body needs.
- To plan. If you know that you will have a very busy schedule in the coming days, why not prepare some meals ahead of time and put them in the freezer?

Three main components make up a slow cooker: the outer shell, the inner food container, and a lid. The outer shell is constructed of metal and contains all the heating coils required for cooking the food, but the coils are built into the outer shell, so they are fully protected. The inner container is referred to as the crock and this is constructed using ceramic that is glazed and fits snugly within the container. There are slow cookers where you can remove the inside container, ideal for when it comes to cleaning it! The final part of the slow cooker is the lid designed to fit perfectly to ensure none of the steam can escape during the cooking process.

So, energize your life and sustain a healthy body by applying what you've discovered. You don't have to change everything at once. Just start by adopting a new recipe each week that sounds interesting to you. Gradually, swap out less-than-healthy options for ingredients and recipes from this book that will promote your well-being.

Each time you make a healthy substitution or try a new ketogenic recipe, you can feel proud of yourself; you are taking good care of your mind and body. Even before you start to experience the benefits of a ketogenic lifestyle, you can feel good because you are choosing the best course for your life.

Thanks for reading.

Lightning Source UK Ltd.
Milton Keynes UK
UKHW020638010621
384722UK00001B/116